YOUR KNOWLEDGE HAS VALUE

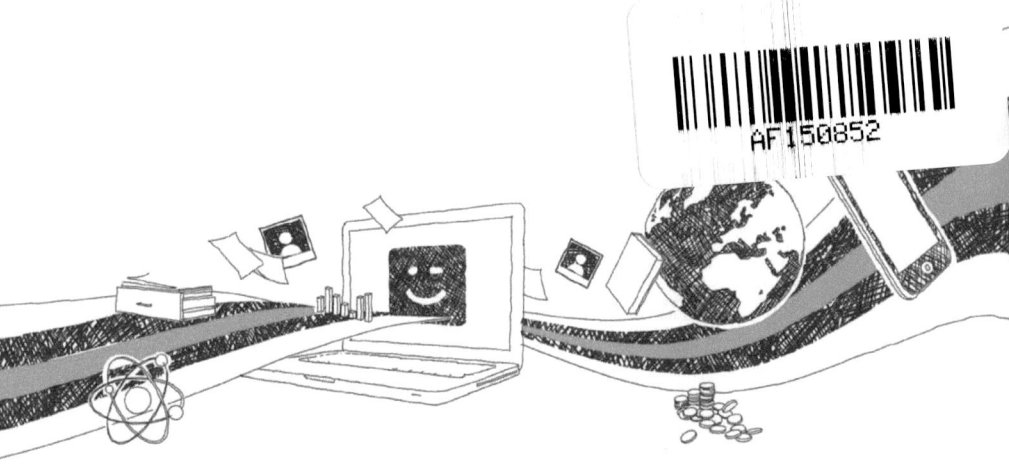

- We will publish your bachelor's and master's thesis, essays and papers

- Your own eBook and book - sold worldwide in all relevant shops

- Earn money with each sale

Upload your text at www.GRIN.com and publish for free

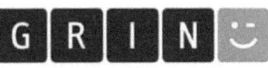

Bibliographic information published by the German National Library:

The German National Library lists this publication in the National Bibliography; detailed bibliographic data are available on the Internet at http://dnb.dnb.de .

Imprint:

Copyright © 2016 GRIN Verlag, Open Publishing GmbH
Print and binding: Books on Demand GmbH, Norderstedt Germany
ISBN: 9783668275850

This book at GRIN:

http://www.grin.com/en/e-book/337556/quality-assurance-in-dental-radiology

Shams Ul Nisa

Quality Assurance in Dental Radiology

GRIN Publishing

GRIN - Your knowledge has value

Since its foundation in 1998, GRIN has specialized in publishing academic texts by students, college teachers and other academics as e-book and printed book. The website www.grin.com is an ideal platform for presenting term papers, final papers, scientific essays, dissertations and specialist books.

Visit us on the internet:

http://www.grin.com/

http://www.facebook.com/grincom

http://www.twitter.com/grin_com

Table of Contents

Quality Assurance In Dental Radiology[1,2, 3,4]

Quality assurance has been defined as the organized effort by staff to ensure the production of high quality radiographs providing consistently adequate diagnostic information at the lowest possible cost and with the least possible exposure of the patient to radiation

An adequate quality radiograph is one, which provides the required diagnostic information. However the quality of radiograph depends upon several contributory factors. Where the practioners is in any doubt about the reasons for poor radiographic quality It is helpful to systematically target the problem areas. This is achieved by carrying out a film reject analysis.

Film Reject Analysis [2]

A subjective evaluation of film quality, which involves keeping a record of radiograph, produced in the practice in particular the poor quality or rejected radiographs.

A simple reject log such as that illustrated below

Film reject Log	Date from .... to					
Log no	Film quality acceptable	Rejected Films				
		Too Dark	Too Pale	Low Contrast	Unsharp image	Poor Positioning
Total						

This reject log kept in the surgery and filled in as the films are viewed will supply a great deal of useful information in a simple and effective manner.

It is sensible to keep separate logs for Dental films and screen films as each has different problems. After an appropriate period of time perhaps after about a hundred films a total numbers are added up to give both an estimate of the reject rate and basic information about the major problems.

Using this possible underlying causes of poor quality can be identified and you can investigate the corrective action using the below information.

Reasons for Rejection

Possible causes   Remedy to Each particular Fault

1. Film too dark
   a) Processing Fault
      - Developer concentration   Dilute or change chemicals
        too High
      - Developing Time too   Adjusted as necessary
        Long
      - Developer temperature   Adjusted as necessary
        Too high

   b) Excessive X-ray exposure
      - Incorrect exposure set   Adjusted and repeat examination
      - Faulty timer of X-ray   Arrange service and repair of faulty
        set   timer of X-ray Set

   c) Fogged Film
      - Light leak in Dark room   Check and correct
      - Faulty safe light   Inspect safe lights visually,
                                     Do Coin test and correct any
                                     Fault detected
      - Old film stock   Discard film
      - Poor film storage   Discard film and reaccess
                                     Storage facility
      - Light leak in cassette   Check hinches and catches
                                     Of cassette and repair or
                                     Replace if required

2. Film too Pale

a) Processing fault
   - Over diluted developer   Change chemicals
   - Inadequate development   Adjust as necessary
     Time
   - Developer temperature   Adjust as necessary
     Too low
   - Exhausted developer   Change chemicals
   - Developer contaminated   Change chemicals
     By fixer

b) Inadequate X-ray Exposure
   - Incorrect exposure set   Adjust and repeat
   - Faulty timer on X-ray set   Arrange service for repair
                                            Of faulty timer of X-ray set

3. Low contrast

a) Processing fault
   - Over development(plus   Check development and
     Dark films)   time/temperature relationship
   - Under development(plus   Check development and
     Pale films)   time/temperature relationship
   - Developer contaminated   Change chemicals
     By fixer
   - Inadequate fixation time   Adjust as necessary
   - Fixer exhaustion   Change Fixer solution

b) Fogged film
   - See above   See above

4. Unsharp Image

     ➤ Patient movement   Assess and instruct
                                              Patients carefully

     ➤ Pure patient positioning   Greater care in
       (In Panoramic radiography)   Positioning with full
                                              use of aids for position-
                                            ning available on equipment

     ➤ Poor Film/Screen contact   Check Hinches and catches of
                                              Cassette and repair or replace if
                                            required.

5. Poor positioning

     ➤ Film incorrectly positioned Use film holders for intra oral
       Or film movement   Radiography when possible

     ➤ X-ray Tube incorrectly   Use film holders with extra oral
       Positioned   beam aiming device attachment

     ➤ Patient incorrectly placed   Greater care in positioning with
       (Panoramic radiography)   full use of aids for positioning
                                            available on equipment.

Solving the Problems[2]

The following areas are targeted when quality of radiographs is tested with reject analysis

➤ Operator Technique

➤ The X-ray Set

➤ The image receptor

➤ The dark room environment and

➤ Processing

Operator Technique [2]

Even with the state of the art X-ray equipment and a perfectly equipped dark room, useless radiographs can still be produced because of poor radiographic technique. The most common and important problems in intra-oral radiographic technique are bending of the film leading to distortion, misdirecting the X-ray beam leading to distortion and overlapping of important areas.

5

'coning off' the film due to incorrect tube position and not maintaining the film in a correct relationship to the area of interest. All these problems can be minimized by using film holders, as recommended in correct guidelines to the profession. The most effective film holders consist of a rigid backing to prevent bending of the film and image distortion .A bite section to ensure the retention of the film packet in the correct position and an extra oral beam aiming device to eliminate coning of and to ensure that the beam is directed correctly.

Periapical Radiography [2,5]

The most practitioners take periapical radiograph using the bisecting angle technique. Inevitably this technique is subject to many errors because of the wide variation in shape and size of mouths and the lack of precision in tube positioning. Various designs of film holders are commercially available but the rinn XCP system of film holders are probably the best known, the system consists of bite blocks, Beam aiming rings and steel connector bars. They are assembled in a number of ways to cope with different areas of mouth.

In the paralleling technique the film is invariably at a greater distance from the teeth than in the bisecting angle technique so a long X-ray source to skin distance is recommended to avoid unacceptable blurring of the image. The 20 cms distance found on all new dental X-ray sets is adequate for this purpose.

Quality standards for periapical radiography [5,6]

A: Evidence of optimal image geometry
- ➢ There should be no evidence of bending of the teeth and the periapical region of interest on the image.
- ➢ There should be no foreshortening or elongation of the teeth.
- ➢ Ideally, there should be no horizontal overlap. If overlap is present, it must not obscure pulp/root canals.

B: Correct anatomical coverage
- ➢ The film should demonstrate all the tooth/teeth of interest (i.e. crown and root[s]).
- ➢ There should be 2-3 mm of periapical bone visible to enable an assessment of apical anatomy.

C: Good density and contrast
- ➢ There should be good density and adequate contrast between the enamel and the dentine.

D: Adequate number of films

➤ In endodontic treatment, it may be necessary to separate superimposed root canals using two radiographs at different horizontal angles. Obtain one 'normal' film and one with a 20 _ oblique horizontal beam angle for all molars and maxillary first premolars.

➤ Assessment of some horizontally impacted mandibular third molars may require two films to image the apex. Obtain one 'normal' film and one with a more posterior 20-degree oblique horizontal beam angle.

E: Adequate processing and darkroom techniques

➤ No pressure marks on film, no emulsion scratches.

➤ No roller marks (automatic processing only).

➤ No evidence of film fog.

➤ No chemical streaks/splashes/contamination.

➤ No evidence of inadequate fixation/washing.

Bite wing Radiography [2,5]

In this accurate orientation of the X-ray beam is essential to avoid the overlap of contact points which reduces information .In addition a consistent X-ray beam orientation is important because it has been demonstrated that the apparent depth of interproximal carious lesions changes significantly with different horizontal angulations. A standardized technique is there for essential for accurate diagnosis and monitoring of caries progression. This can be achieved by using special bitewing film holders incorporating the features described.

Quality standards for bitewing radiography [5,6]

A: Evidence of optimal image geometry

➤ There should be no evidence of bending of the teeth and the periapical region of interest on the image.

➤ There should be no foreshortening or elongation of the teeth.

➤ Ideally, there should be no horizontal overlap. If overlap is present, it must not obscure pulp/root canals.

B: Correct anatomical coverage

➤ The film should demonstrate all the tooth/teeth of interest (i.e. crown and root[s]).

➤ There should be 2-3 mm of periapical bone visible to enable an assessment of apical anatomy.

C: Good density and contrast

➤ There should be good density and adequate contrast between the enamel and the dentine.

D: Adequate number of films

➤ In endodontic treatment, it may be necessary to separate superimposed root canals using two radiographs at different horizontal angles. Obtain one 'normal' film and one with a 20 _ oblique horizontal beam angle for all molars and maxillary first premolars.

➤ Assessment of some horizontally impacted mandibular third molars may require two films to image the apex. Obtain one 'normal' film and one with a more posterior 20 _ oblique horizontal beam angle.

E: Adequate processing and darkroom techniques

➤ No pressure marks on film, no emulsion scratches.

➤ No roller marks (automatic processing only).

➤ No evidence of film fog.

➤ No chemical streaks/splashes/contamination.

➤ No evidence of inadequate fixation/washing.

Panoramic Radiography [2,5]

Poor positioning will cause blurring and distortion of the teeth. In addition to correct positioning with respect to the focal plane the patient must be in an erect posture with shoulders back and neck straight to avoid a pronounced midline image of the cervical spine.

All metallic objects from around the head and neck, which would be in the line of X-ray beam, should be moved. Earrings, Hearing aids, Necklaces, Dentures and spectacles can all produce primary and secondary images, which obscure important information

Panoramic radiograph involve long exposure times typically fifteen to twenty seconds .So it is essential that movement is avoided to prevent the production of misleading images on the films. Consequently patients whose cooperation is in doubt should be carefully instructed before taking the X-ray

Quality standards for panoramic radiography [5,6]

A: Patient preparation/ instruction adequate

➤ Edge to edge incisors.

➤ No removable metallic foreign bodies (e.g. earrings, spectacles, dentures).

➤ No motion artifacts.

> Tongue against roof of mouth.

> Minimization of spine shadow.

B: No patient positioning errors

> No antero-posterior positioning errors (equal vertical and horizontal magnification).

> No mid sagittal plane positioning errors (symmetrical magnification).

> No occlusal plane positioning errors.

> Correct positioning of spinal column.

C: Correct anatomical coverage

> Appropriate coverage depending upon the clinical application. Field size limitation should have been used (if available) to exclude structures irrelevant to clinical needs (e.g. limitation of field to teeth and alveolar bone for everyday dental use).

D: Good density and contrast

> There should be good density and adequate contrast between the enamel and the dentine.

E: No cassette/ screen problems

> No light leaks.

> Good film/screen contact.

> Clean screens.

F: Adequate processing and darkroom techniques

> No pressure marks on film, no emulsion scratches.

> No roller marks (automatic processing only).

> No evidence of film fog.

> No chemical streaks/splashes/contamination.

> No evidence of inadequate fixation/washing.

> Name/date/left or right marker all legible.

Cephalometric radiography [2,5]

It is intrinsic to the purposes of Cephalometric radiography that images are reproducible. This requires a fixed X-ray source/patient/image receptor relationship. It is unacceptable to perform Cephalometric radiography without a cephalostat to fix head position. Most dentists working in primary dental care would use an integrated Panoramic/Cephalometric radiographic system. However, some may use a dental X-ray set as the source. The large distance of patient to X-ray source required in cephalometry, is such that using an unmodified dental X-ray set would lead to an unacceptably large X-ray field and excessive radiation dose. Therefore, dental

X-ray equipment must be suitably modified to ensure correct collimation and alignment by direct involvement of a medical physics expert.

Quality standards for Cephalometric radiography [5,6]

A: Patient preparation/ instruction adequate

➤ Frankfort plane perpendicular to film.

➤ No sagittal plane positioning errors.

➤ No occlusal plane positioning errors

➤ Teeth in centric occlusion (stable and natural intercuspation).

➤ Lips relaxed.

B: No patient positioning errors

➤ No antero-posterior positioning errors.

➤ No mid sagittal plane positioning errors.

➤ No occlusal plane positioning errors.

➤ Exact matching of external auditory meatus with positioning devices.

C: Correct anatomical coverage

➤ Visibility of all Cephalometric tracing points required for the analysis.

➤ Visibility of all anterior skeletal and soft tissue structures.

D: Good density and contrast

E: No cassette/ screen problems

➤ No light leaks.

➤ Good film/screen contact.

➤ Clean screens.

F: Adequate processing and darkroom techniques

➤ No evidence of film fog.

➤ No evidence of chemical streaks/contamination.

➤ No evidence of inadequate fixation /washing.

➤ No evidence of screen damage/artifacts.

➤ No roller marks/pressure marks.

➤ Name and date legible.

The X-ray Set [2]

Quality assurance of the X-ray set involves three areas of importance. Radiation safety, Mechanical stability and function (ie the movement of the arm and tube head, the intactness of the tube head casing and the control panel/handset and the rigidity of the attachment of the collimator cylinder to the tube head) and electrical safety and function (i.e. How well the components work and the accuracy of the calibration of the Kilo watts, Milli amperes and the timer). The dentist can carry out simple visual inspection of the cable and plug and also identify any drift of the tube/arm after positioning for clinical use.

Radiation safety should include checks on filtration, beam alignment and collimation, Kilo Voltage and exposure. Adherence to current statutory regulations, which requires a radiation survey of X-ray equipment once every 3 years helps to ensure that safety, is maintained.

The dental monitoring service postal pack currently available from the national radiological protection board fulfills these statutory requirements for the radiation safety survey.

The regulation also indicates that regular servicing and maintenance of the mechanical and electrical aspect of X-ray equipment should be instituted at intervals recommended by the manufacturer.

Good radiographic technique is essential for high quality images, but the procedures carried out before and after the exposure are of equal importance. These procedures, which are called collectively "radiographic photography", need to be followed in an exacting way and with at least a basic understanding of the nature of the material and equipment.

One factor of obvious importance in radiography is that the image receptors are stored and handled properly and this will be considered first.

The Image Receptor [3, 6, 7]

Film

Two basic types of films are used in radiography.

➢ The film used in cassettes which is manufactured to be optimally sensitive to the light emitted from the intensifying screens when the latter are exposed to X-rays

➢ Dental and occlusal film ('non screen film') which is designed to be optimally sensitive to X-rays.

Ideally all film should be stored under cool and dry conditions. Temperatures should not exceed 21degress or 'fogging' of films (an increase in overall film density leading to dark radiograph with reduced contrast) will result .in addition, all film should be used before its expiry date because old film is likely to become fogged. Shelf life can be extended considerably by storage in a refrigerator but only if the packets of films are unopened to avoid moisture contamination.

Environmental contaminants can adversely affect the film. The most obvious potential contaminants are X-rays and common sense dictates keeping films as far from the X-ray source as possible. In practice, however, it is usually convenient to keep films close to X-ray set and suitable containers are available which offer protection against radiation.

Visible light is not a problem for dental or occlusal films unless the protective film packet is damaged leading to perforation contamination. However screen films can easily be exposed to light if the lid of film box is left off. This typically exposes just one edge of the film leading to a characteristic pattern of fogging. The consequences of spoiling a full box of film can be avoided by transferring enough films in the darkroom into a second box to deal with a typical day's workload.

The emulsion of film is sensitive to mechanical damage. Bending of films during radiography or in darkroom may lead to artifacts on the processed radiographs. Consequently film should be handled as gently as possible.

Discharges of static electricity are an uncommon but irritating problem occurring more frequently with larger screen films than dental films. the cause of static discharge can be difficult to identify but the phenomena appears to be more common in warm dry atmosphere.

Intensifying screens and cassettes [3,6]

As the radiographic image on screen film is produced by emission of light which occurs from the intensifying screens when they are exposed to X-rays, anything which prevents that light from reaching the film will result in artifacts and reduce overall film quality .It is therefore essential that the screen surfaces should be kept clean and free from contamination by dust, grime and foreign material .The risk can also be reduced by only opening screens when films are being loaded or unloaded from the cassette .In addition the screens should be cleaned regularly using a proprietary screen cleaner with a clean soft and dry cloth.

Many different intensifying screens are manufactured for radiography. These differ in various ways for example in 'speed'. However, there are two principle types. The traditional calcium tungstate screens and the newer, faster rare earth screens. The former emit a blue light while most of the latter emit a green light. As a result the film used must be matched to the screens a mismatch will result in a pale, low contrast radiograph.

When more than one cassette of a particular type is used in the dental practice it is worthwhile marking the cassettes. This can be done by either fixing lead numbers to the cassette or marking one of the screens in each cassette with a pen. If an artefact or fault is seen on the radiograph then the cassette involved can then be quickly identified and corrected.

Light leakage into cassette results in film fogging and poor film / screen contact leads to blurred image. Both these faults are usually caused by incompletely closing the cassette. However a faulty or damaged hinge may cause these problems to recur.

The Darkroom.[3,6,8]

Every effort must be made to prevent exposure of the film emulsion to the daylight or ordinary artificial lighting if film fogging is to be avoided .It should be noted that any deficiency in darkroom condition will have more deleterious effects on screen films than on dental films because the former is more sensitive to light. Consequently a practioner who finds that panaromic and other screen films are dark with low contrast while the dental films are satisfactory should check light-tightness and safe lighting of the darkroom.

It should be noted that different film types. For example films sensitive to rare earth screen light emissions and those sensitive to calcium tungstate screen light emissions may require different safelight conditions .It is important to check the manufacturer's recommendation for the type of safelight filter required, particularly when changing your film supplier or manufacturer.

Light tightness must be tested before considering the safelights .The simplest way to check is to stand in the darkroom with door closed and the safelights turned off and inspect visually for signs of daylight. It is important to allow at least a minute for the eyes to accommodate in the darkness before checking. Light leaks can then be marked on the walls or around the door using chalk or another suitable marker to permit identification after the lights are turned on.

Once it has been established that the darkroom is light- tight the safe lighting must be checked. Basic safe lighting rules should be adhered to. Filters should be inspected regularly to check for crackage or other deterioration. If the safelight appears satisfactory then a simple 'coin' test should be carried out to assess how safe the lighting is. This entails placing a coin (or another opaque object) on a piece of screen film (or an unwrapped dental film) in the darkroom with safelights turned on. This is left for approximately a minute film then processed normally. Fogging of film due to poor safe lighting will then be obvious because of the clear area left where the coin protected the film from the light. It may be useful to gradually expose a film with a number of coins on to a given range of times of exposure to safelights .In practice the crucial time for which the safelights must not fog for films and be normal handling the time of films before processing and this may vary from few seconds up to a minute or more when the dental surgery assistant is loading a film hanger with a dozen dental films.

Coin test should always be carried out on the screen films, unless only dental films are used in the dental practice, because of the greater light sensitivity.

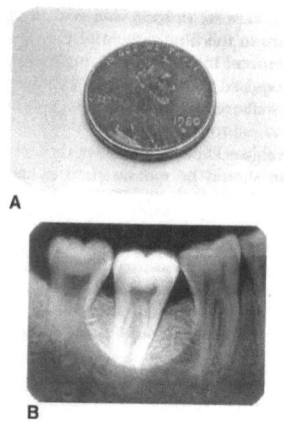

Coin Test for unsafe illumination

Cleanliness[3]

Precisely because a darkroom is dark, contamination of films with chemical splashes and damp fingers is easy. This can be prevented by cleaning the work surfaces daily and immediately during spillage or splashes. Chemicals should be stored well away from the work surfaces, Where processing is carried out physically, film hangers should be cleaned to prevent accumulated chemical residues producing streak artefacts on films.

Processing[3]

Optimal processing is of paramount importance in ensuring high quality radiographs. Unfortunately .The Dental Monitoring Services of NRPB has revealed that X-ray exposure is often increased to compensate for inadequate development.

Despite the supposed superiority of automatic processors in removing the possible variables of manual processing, the NRPB survey shown that 30% of practices with automatic processors were using a radiographic exposure 50% greater than the considered necessary for optimum quality radiographs. This appears to be due to a combination of incorrect operation, inadequate maintenance and lack of attention to renewal and preparation of processing solutions.

Manual Processing[3]

Attention to basic details should help to reduce unsatisfactory processing. The general points to be noted are as follows.

➤ An accurate thermometer and timer are essential in the darkroom. The timer should have a second hand for accuracy.

➤ Solution levels should be checked and topped up when necessary to avoid insufficient coverage of the films during processing.

➤ Solutions should be stirred prior to use to ensure even temperatures in the tanks.

➤ Films should be occasionally agitated during processing to bring fresh chemicals into contact with the emulsion and to displace any attached air bubbles

➤ Chemicals tanks should have lids to reduce evaporation.to limit developer oxidation and to avoid contamination.

Development[3]

Correct development depends upon the proper concentration of developer solution being used at the correct temperature for the specified time. Underdevelopment due to over diluted or exhausted developer, low temperatures and /or inadequate time will produce radiographs lacking in density and contrast. Overdevelopment due to insufficiently diluted developer, high temperature and/or excessive time will produce radiograph which are not only too dark but which also have a high chemical 'fog' level; the latter being due to development of unexposed crystals in emulsion.

Thus attention to the manufactures instruction for dilution of developer concentrate and to temperature/time relationship is essential. It is the responsibility of the dentist to emphasize the importance of these factors to the DSA who is responsible for the processing.

Developer is a reducing agent and oxidizes in contact with air until its potency is ultimately lost. Developer solution should be changed at least once every four weeks and preferably once every 10-14 days if underdevelopment is to be avoided.

Wash[3]

Washing the films briefly between development and fixation avoids contamination of the acid fixer by alkaline developer. Failure to include this stage will shorten the life of the fixer solution.

Fixation[3]

Fixer removes unexposed grains of emulsion. Visually this manifests in the 'clearing' of the films, with the gradual emergence of an image from the previously opaque film. Fixation is not dependant significantly upon the temperature. However an adequate time for fixation is important. Too short a time will leave areas of opacity on the radiograph, which will be visible on viewing by transmitted light. These areas obscure detail and discolor with time. The films should remain in the fixer for at least twice the development time.

Second wash[3]

This is important to remove the fixer completely from the film. Failure to carry this out will cause a characteristic brownish discoloration to develop. Ideally films should be washed in running water for 30 minutes. Ofcourse, if a radiograph is urgently required in surgery the wash can be briefly postponed. However the film should be returned for completion of washing directly after inspection.

Drying[3]

Before either mounting or storing films they should be quiet dry. Damp films will stick to each other or to the paper of envelopes with risk of damaging the still fairly delicate gelatin surface of radiograph. Drying cabinets can be purchased but are not essentials; simply allowing the films to dry in air while attached to film hangers is satisfactory; an electric fan can be used to speed up the drying process.

Automatic Processing [3,6]

Many dental practices now use automatic processing equipments. Their use can remove many of variables from processing radiographs but consistent and correct result depends on maintenance of the equipment. Processors should be serviced at intervals recommended by the manufacturer. The chemical and wash tanks should be drained and cleaned weekly to remove residues and prevent growth of algae. Where the processors use a roller transport system, the rollers should be removed and cleaned at the same time. Passing a trial film (cleaner) through the rollers in the morning before clinical use will also help remove dried chemical residues, which would otherwise be transferred onto clinical radiographs.

Monitoring Radiographic Processing

There is value in processing a test radiograph once a day and visually comparing it with a standard reference film to check the consistency of film quality. If you tend to process your radiographs in bulk at the end of the day then the test films should be processed immediately before the clinical films after preparation of chemicals. If it is usual to process films as and when they are taken then test film should be processed daily, at the same time each day. The reference film should be prepared when the chemicals are changed under carefully controlled development time and temperature conditions.

A new reference film should be prepared each time chemicals are renewed.

A clinical film, for example a bitewing produced on the day chemicals were changed, can be used as reference films. Bitewings produced on subsequent day can act as test films. However this is open to criticism because of the wide variation between different patients. it is far better to take radiograph of some standard object each day and use this as the monitoring film. In the USA quality assurance test objects can be acquired for the dental practice. Unfortunately this is not readily available and the alternatives usually have to be sought. An extracted tooth or teeth can be used for this purpose. It should be noted that when taking the test radiographs the same exposure conditions must always be used, including a consistent distance between the X-ray source and the film and the same orientation on the film.

The ideal standard object is one which gives image with wide variation in film density and contrast and which facilitates visual comparison of test and reference films. Traditionally a stepped wedge phantom constructed of aluminium is used, but a perfectly adequate substitute can be prepared using materials found in the dental practice. For example, four pieces of lead foil found in dental film packets can be arranged 'stepwise' to mimic the stepped wedge phantom and stuck to a piece of card or plastic with adhesive tape. Use the normal exposure time for a bitewing radiograph when exposing the stepped wedge. Simple visual comparison of reference and test films can detect changes in film quality before gross deterioration occurs.

Processing variables have a more noticeable affect on the quality of screen films than on dental films. Consequently there is a greater need for monitoring in practices using screen films. Where automatic processors are used monitoring films is also of value. in larger practices, where expensive automatic processors are installed and radiographic workload is high there may be a need for a more objective and sophisticated form of processor monitoring.

References:

1. **Enrique Platin et al**, A quantitative analysis of dental radiography quality assurance practices among North Carolena dentists, Oral surgery, Oral medicine ,Oral pathology ,Oral radiology, Endodontics, 1998, 86 : 115 – 120

2. **K.Horner**, Quality assurance : 1 .Reject analysis, Operator technique and the x-ray set , Dental update, March 1992, 75 – 80

3. **K.Horner**, Quality assurance : 2 .The image receptor ,the dark room and processing , Dental update ,April 1992, 120 – 126

4. **James Rgeist et al** ,Radiation dose – reduction techniques in North American dental schools, Oral surgery ,Oral medicine, Oral Pathalogy, Oral Radiology, Endodontics 2002 ;93 : 496 – 505

5. **European guidelines on radiation protection in dental radiology** , 136, 2004

6. **White and Pharoah** ,Text book of Oral Radiology ,Principles and interpretation ,5th edition

7. **Peter.N.Hirsehmann** , Dose limitation in dental radiography ,Dental update ,July 1993 ,257 – 261

8. **AERB** ,Safety code for medical diagnostic x-ray equipment and installations, October 5 , 2001

YOUR KNOWLEDGE HAS VALUE

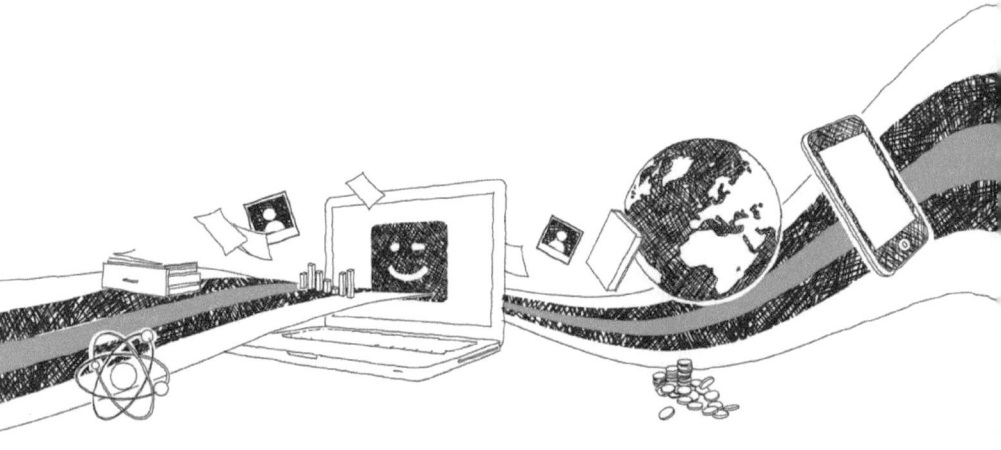

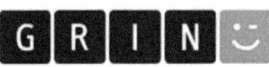